The Agili Wellness Routine, Book 1

By

Ofer Agam

ISBN: 1-4140-0444-3 (e-book)
ISBN: 1-4140-0445-1 (Paperback)

This book is printed on acid free paper.

Photography by Howard Scheiman.

1stBooks - rev. 01/08/04

A Disclaimer

If you have a chronic illness, or suffer from an injury, or just want to improve your daily life, you owe it to yourself to incorporate all, or parts of the Agili Wellness Routine into your life. But you must also share this book with a physician who is familiar with your state of health, in order to make sure that stretches and exercises mentioned in this book are appropriate and safe for you to use. I would hate to see you hurt yourself while using this routine or advice, and will not take any responsibility if you do. Start slowly and examine each option presented carefully, before and as you perform it.

To my wife Nitza, and my children, David and Ori.

Introduction

My first symptoms of MS occurred in April 1974, when I was 19 years old; my heels were buzzing with a constant tingling sensation. No one knew what I had, but I was told to rest and relax, which was not a very realistic form of therapy for a normal young adult. In my case, it was a relief, since by then and for a long while I had had to function as a soldier in spite of great fatigue. In 1980, two years after I came from Israel to the San Francisco Bay Area, I was stricken with optic neuritis. My ophthalmologist sent me to a neurologist. "Just to make sure you're fine," he assured me on my way out of his office, after I failed to count fingers on his raised hand from three feet away.

The neurologist, a gentleman, didn't think I had MS. "What's MS?" I asked, and couldn't hide the faint alarm that came out with my quick response. "Oh, well," he said as he guided me to a comfortable chair. "Why don't you sit down for a moment, and tell me a little about yourself?"

"I go to City College," I started, feeling a bit more relaxed. "I'm trying to get a certificate in computer programming, but I'm very tired, and stopped driving—at least for now."

"In most cases, eye sight problems get better over time," he explained, and then listened patiently as I told him about my upbringing and military service.

"What do you do first thing in the morning?" The neurologist surprised me with a smile on his face.

"I don't know," I hesitated. "I take a shower?"

"Shower, yes," he quickly responded. "Do you use hot water?"

"Sometimes…" I paused for a moment. "Sometimes, when I bend my head down after a shower, you know, to pick up a towel from the floor…"

"Yes…"

"Well, I feel this shock from my neck all the way down to my tail bone…" The man couldn't hide his disappointment. He then took about 10 minutes to gently explain to me what was years later confirmed with MRI. Two days later, when I excitedly announced to the neurologist over the phone that I was going to New York to treat my MS with injections of snake venom, he quickly referred me to a research neurologist up at the VA hospital in San Francisco, and had me promise that I would cancel my trip to New York.

Since then, I sought healing in many ways, including gluten-free and other diets, massive amounts of food supplements, drugs such as Baclofen, Zanaflex and IV steroids. Scientists are now testing statins with promising results for immune modulation, and I am taking Zocor with my doctor's supervision. I tried physical therapy and other physical methods and techniques. I bought exercise machines that I still try and use as often as I can, but none helped me as much as my own home-grown relaxing, stretching and exercise routine.

It all started when I once accompanied a friend on his way to his daily exercise. I was going to wait for him on the beach and read the paper during his run.

"What's the benefit of this?" I asked when I saw him lifting one leg over the concrete rail.

"Without using this stretch, I can't run much," he said pulling on his elevated foot. "It greatly reduces my lower back pain…" He added, "I use it before and after my run."

I have lower back pain, I thought to myself, *and sometimes I can't walk much at all when it's bad. But how am I going to put my leg up on some fence?*

This turned out to be a transforming event for me. Once I figured out how to stretch my legs without the rail, and reduce my lower back discomfort to negligible levels, I started walking a little better and exercising a little longer. Over a period of few years, I reached the conclusion that exercising while lying on one's back both greatly reduces the risk of injury and yet can be very effective, even for aerobics. I realized that progress, however small it may seem, leads to great benefits. I learned that I needed to continue to use and improve my routine every day, because it made me more agile. It had the wonderful cumulative effect of slowly regaining function taken away from me by illness.

For some, this routine will work very quickly, and they will feel better and less tight right away. For others, it may take a bit longer to notice a great difference, but all will benefit from using this system of very effective stretches and exercises. With your gained agility, you will prevent or reduce accidents such as falling or bumping into different objects. Your ankles will slowly get stronger, your grip will improve and stamina increase. All, no matter how dire their situations may seem, can improve!

Mine is a pragmatic approach, and a solution to a real problem: how to become more agile in the face of muscular issues. Increasing one's flexibility and range of motion goes a very long way towards improving one's life. I am not expecting you to contort your body into some kind of submission. Instead, I am suggesting that you lie down on your back, meditate for a while, and then gently and gradually stretch your main muscle groups and joints. As you get stronger, perform the exercises presented and increase your aerobic stamina as well. It is not only people with illness who experience muscular degeneration, and many suffer debilitating back pain—but not enough to be labeled "handicapped". If you are an athlete, use the stretches before your run or game. You will hit the ball farther, dribble better, or kick it more accurately. Try my Agili Wellness Routine, and you will be more alert, more nimble, and less tired. Your mood will improve, and you will feel a new and positive energy that will accompany you wherever you go. The more you practice it, the more empowered you will feel.

Stretches and exercises are most effective when enough time is dedicated to each. If your joints or muscles or any part of your body is hurting, it means that you are overextending your body. Stop, and try the stretch or exercise later. Over time, the pain will be replaced with a pleasant and addictive agility that comes after you finish your Agili Wellness Routine.

Too much: too much, is by definition, too much. We each have a margin, over which we should not go; an invisible line that warns us of an injury or a pending setback to our health. Use common sense before and during your Agili Wellness Routine.

It is best to review the entire book before you start using the Agili Wellness Routine, because some answers to your questions are provided as you go. After you learn how to use the different options presented, select your favorites, and develop a routine that best suits you. I will first explain how to get into an ideal position for meditation, and some good stretches and exercises. We will later move to exercises on your knees and feet for more demanding and aerobic exercises. Finally, I will show you how to cool down and gently end your daily session.

Table of Contents

Some Helpful Accessories

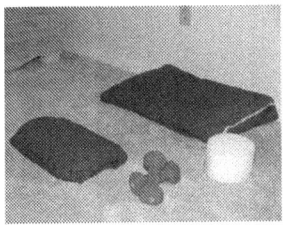

I highly recommend that before you start the Agili Wellness Routine, you equip yourself with the following:

- One pad, placed flush with a smooth and clear wall or sturdy closet. This pad can be a flat and preferably firm pillow or a folded thin blanket.
- One small pillow. Place the pillow so that when you lie down on your back, your bottom will rest on the pad, and your head on the small pillow. Use a small pillow to allow better arm movement around your head.
- One wedge. Another small pillow will do. I cut this wedge from a physical therapy roll that I purchased in a medical supply store.
- Two free weights. You may also use any other object in your household (such as food cans). These are used primarily to stretch your arms and hands.
- A pair of socks to wear during the routine.

You may choose not to use the pad and pillow, but my experience is that it is better to slightly elevate your pelvis and head during the Agili Wellness Routine.

Get on Your Back

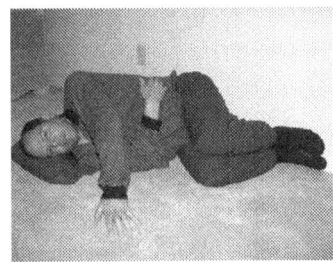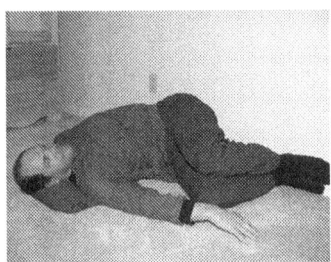

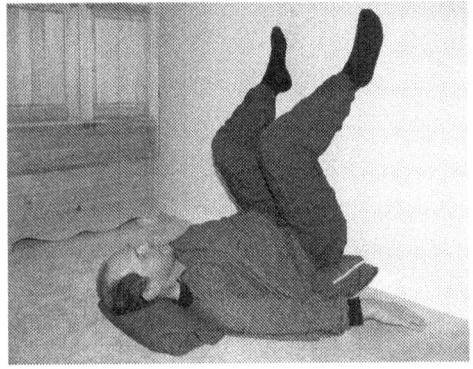

- Before you can start the Agili Wellness Routine, you need to get into position: sit down with your back next to the pad and your side as close to the wall as possible. Lie down on your side, and rest your head on the small pillow, and scoot over to the wall a little more.
- Rotate your body onto your back. (You may choose to stay like this for a few moments if you like the stretch…)
- Lift your legs up and rest your feet on the wall! You are now ready to start. If you find that getting in position is too difficult at first, you may need help from someone else. All positions and exercises in this book are done with the support of a wall or sturdy closet. As you get stronger, this routine will become easier for you to perform. The key to success is to practice every day.

Some Meditation, First

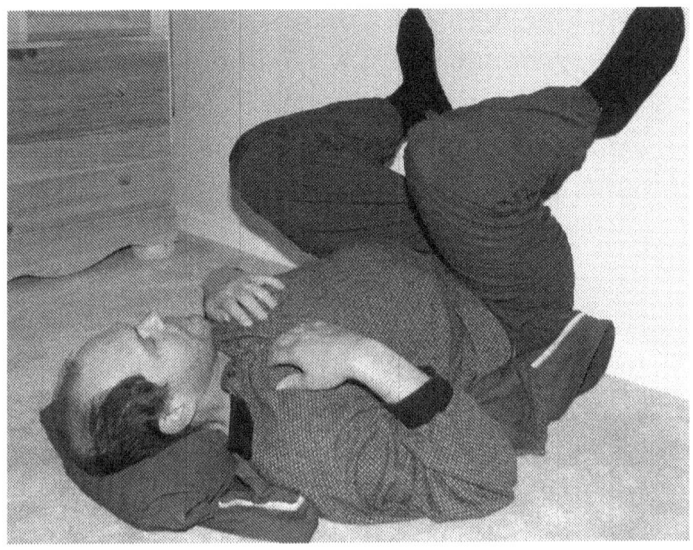

I start my routine squatting on the wall for about 10 minutes. I let my feet fall down the wall, and when they stop, I pull them down a little further with my hands, and end up with my feet flat on the wall. If they don't end up flat, or if you have problems with your knees, do not force your feet down, or flat on the wall. You should feel a pleasant opening pull on muscles around your pelvis, hip joints and lower back. Some of you may be more comfortable crossing your legs in a lotus position; try and see what works best for you.

I place my left hand around my heart, relax my forehead and eyes, and drop my jaw. I take one big breath into my chest and hold it for a few seconds. I then release the air slowly through my mouth with my lips puckered. After this initial preparation, I continue and breathe with focus, and gently raise my stomach as I go. Over years of doing this, I found that it is most relaxing to just be aware and focus on my breathing and not try to exhale longer or inhale deeper. Your mind may wander for a while, but with practice you will be able to extend your focus period, and therefore reach deeper levels of relaxation. It is perfectly fine, if you end up sleeping in this position for a while.

Stretching

Stretching Your Legs:

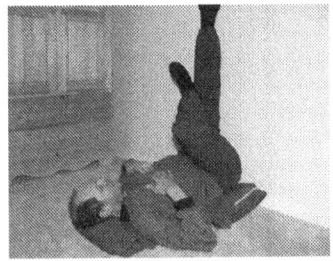 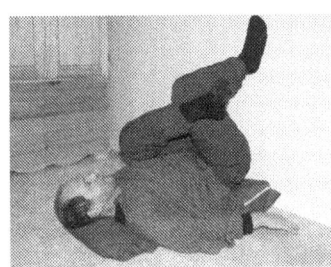

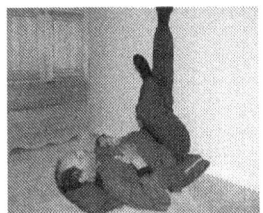

This is a good warm up for more advanced leg stretches

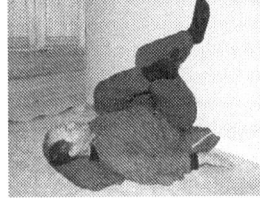

- Put one leg stretched up on the wall, and rest the other on it, just below the knee, as shown in top left picture. You should feel a pleasant stretch in the back of your leg. Remain in this position for a few moments, and then switch legs. To increase your leg stretch, remain close to the wall, but move the pad under the arch of your back, and let your tail bone drop towards the floor behind the pad.
- With one leg still rested below your knee, slide your foot down on the wall and bend your knee. Remain like this a few moments, for each leg.

More Advanced Stretching for Your Legs:

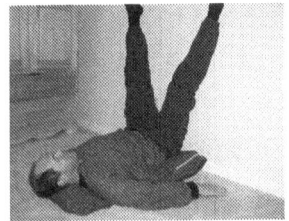 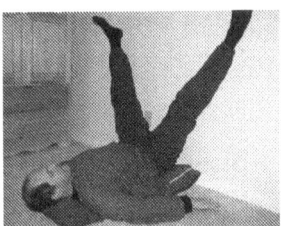

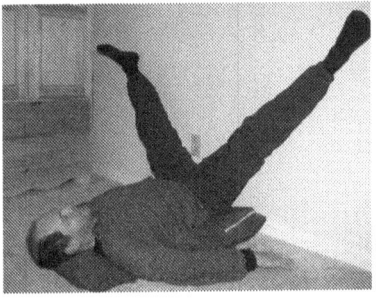

Be aware of your body: to avoid muscle atrophy, if you are using one hand more than the other, make a point of using both. For instance, if you use a computer mouse with your right hand often, use a squeeze ball with the other. As you walk, instead of quickly stepping with your weaker leg, try and spend the same amount of time on each leg.

This stretch is very effective for anyone with lower back pain. Perform this leg stretch as part of your Agili Wellness Routine, or before and after a physical activity.

- Get as close to the wall as possible.
- Push your feet up the wall as far as they will go.
- Spread them apart as far as they will go; let them stop by themselves, and do not stretch your inner thigh beyond comfort.

- Maintain this position for a few moments. Every time you perform it, you will find that this exercise increases your flexibility and lower back health.
- To increase your leg stretch, remain close to the wall, but move the pad up under the arch of your back, and let your tail bone drop towards the floor behind the pad.
- The next day, try to increase the spread...

Loosen Up Your Hip Joints and Thighs:

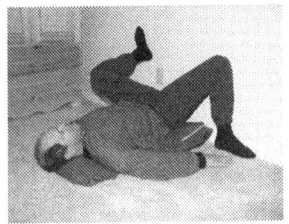 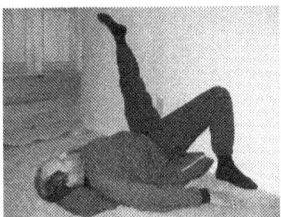

- Lower one foot to the floor, and place it with the knee flush against the wall. Some of you may need to roll sideways a bit to be able to place your foot on the floor and against the wall first, and then rotate back to position. If it is too difficult to put your foot all the way down on the floor, place it higher on the wall.
- Place the other foot, with bent knee, on the wall. Over time, you will be able to increase the spread between your legs.
- After a few moments, stretch your leg up on wall.
- Switch sides.

During this and other stretches, you will discover some new "sleepy" areas in your body. Remain on your back, and massage the sore spots.

A word about self-massage: self-massage is amazingly helpful and contributes to the release of tight muscles. You know best where it hurts, and how a stiff area negatively affects writing or walking, so help yourself with self-massage.

Stretching Your Arms and Hands:

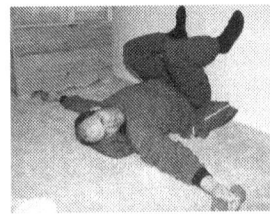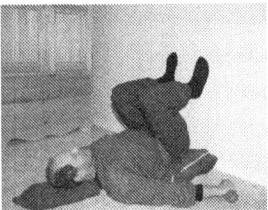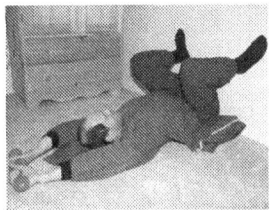

During all legs stretches, it is also a good time to stretch your arms and hands.

- First, with weights in your hands, simply allow your arms to "melt" into the floor. You should feel a mild stretch in your arms and hands.
- Roll the weights to the tip of your fingers and then close your hands on them again.
- Move your arms up and down against the floor, and find the best spot for a good stretch. Stretching your arms and hands will restore agility, flexibility and strength over time.
- Slowly roll your head to one side, and then to the other. Stretching your neck and shoulders will reduce your headaches and can loosen up your entire body.

These are passive stretches. If you need to, use heavier weights to help stretch your hands and arms down to the floor.

A word about your abdomen: your mid-section supports your whole body and enables you maintain a healthy posture. When your abdomen is strong, your lower back is healthier as well, and your agility increases.

To exercise your abdomen and lower back at any time while on your back, with weights, lift your hands off the floor and keep them hovering for a while. Keep your lower back flush with the pad at the same time. To increase difficulty, keep your arms straight, and lift them up, all the way to the floor above your head and back down a number of times.

Exercise on Your Back

After meditating and stretching, you can enjoy some exercises to regain strength and agility. If it works for you, put some music on to help you establish a rhythm suitable for you. Pace yourself, and increase the amount of time you spend with each exercise over time.

Gains from repetition: the more you repeat meditation, the more you will be able to relax, focus and concentrate; even your sleep will improve. The more you repeat stretching, the looser and less tight or spastic you are going to be. The more you repeat exercising, the stronger you will become. Repeat all three, and you will allow energy to flow through your mind and body better, and a sense of well being will envelope you throughout your day.

Up and Down:

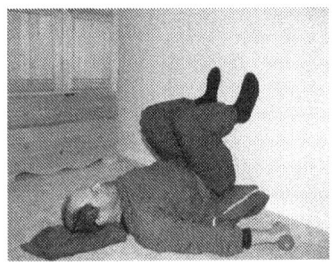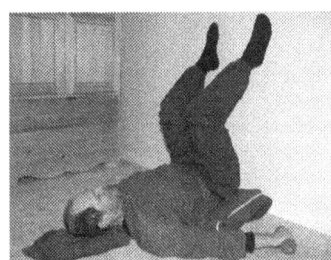

Start moving your feet up and down against the wall. As you get stronger, you can increase the difficulty of this exercise in the following ways:

- Increase the pace of exercise (it is important to try and keep motion identical on both sides, even if it means lower speed).
- Increase friction: the harder you press your feet against the wall, the more energy it takes to continue the motion.
- On your toes: to strengthen your foot, lift your heels off the wall, and perform exercise on your toes.
- On your heels: lift your toes off the wall, and perform exercise with your heels against the wall.

Up and Down with Wedge:

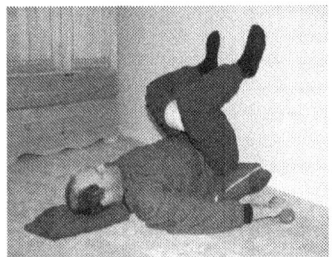 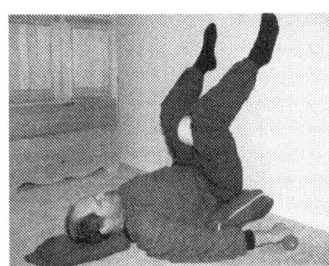

With a wedge or small pillow between your knees, move your feet up and down against the wall. The wedge helps stabilize your legs and allows you to move them together better. Pressing your knees against the wedge is another way to strengthen your legs. As you get stronger, you can increase the difficulty of this exercise as described above.

Up and Down with Hands Pressed Together:

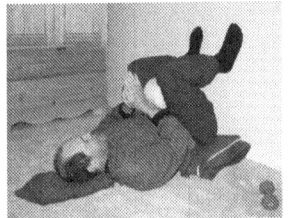 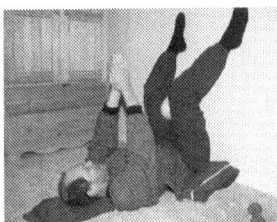

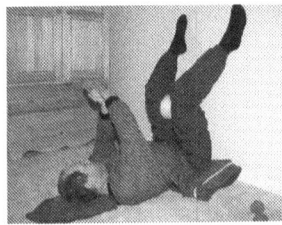

This is a very effective exercise, and can be performed with or without exercising your legs.

- Put your hands together, and match fingers from both hands as best you can.
- Move your hands—slowly and with control—away from your chest all the way up, and then slowly back down.
- Increase pressure on hands to increase difficulty.

You should feel your arms, chest and hands muscles all at the same time. Perform exercise with different hand positions. Put clasped hands over your forehead with your elbows bent, and then move them up and away from your forehead—or try bending one wrist with the other extended as you go up and down.

Up and Down with Weights:

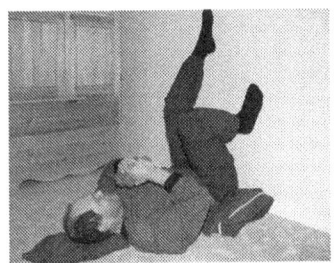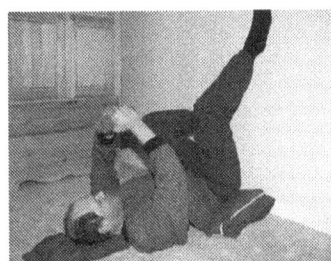

This is an aerobic option that you can choose. As you slide your feet up and down on the wall with a weight in each hand, push your hands away from your chest, and bring them back. To increase hand and arm control and co-ordination, separate your hands and try to lift each with the same leg or opposite leg as you go.

Circular Motion:

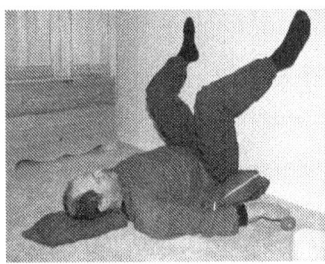 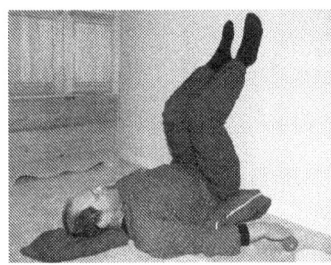

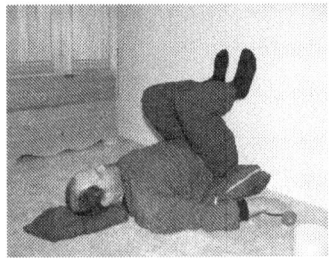 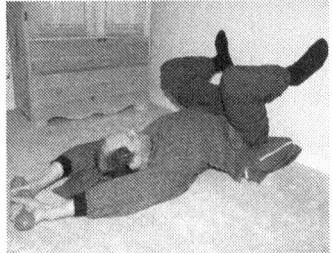

This exercise increases foot and leg control and co-ordination. Still on your back, start a circular motion with both feet against the wall. If you can, rhythmically move your arms and hands with or without weights. Otherwise, take advantage of the time and stretch your arms and hands during the circular motion on the wall. Try exercising your abdomen, or simply rest your arms.

Exercise on Knees

To add variety and challenge to your daily Agili Wellness Routine, exercise on your knees. It may work better for you if you wear a pair of wool gloves or socks on your hands.

Flat Hands:

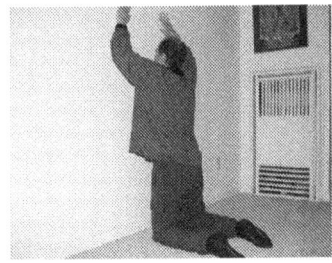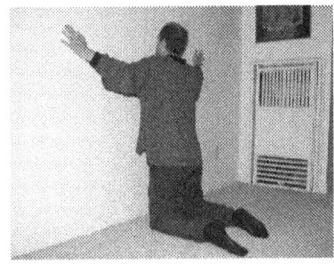

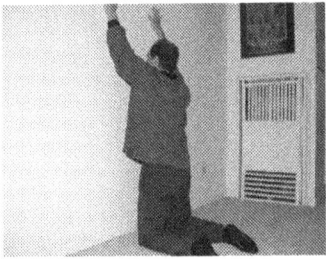

This will not only strengthen your arms, hands, abdomen and back, but if you keep it up for a while, you'll get a very good aerobic workout out of it.

Fisted Hands:

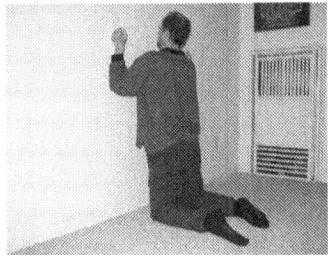 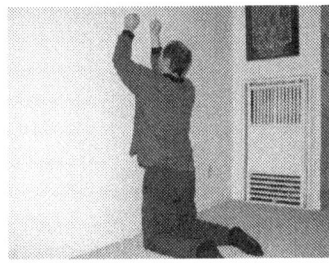

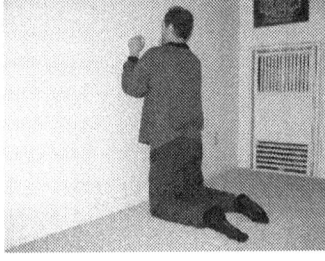

Try and use fisted hands in a circular motion, up and down or sideways.

Exercise on Feet

The most demanding part of the Agili Wellness Routine is done on your feet.

The next day: use the following day to gauge how well you have done. If you walk a little better or pick up a grocery bag without giving it much thought, you are doing great; your Agili pace was good. But if you feel stiff, and walking is more difficult, take a day off from exercising on your knees and feet, and avoid exacerbating your condition. Be patient and allow the time it takes to break down a process that started in your body a long time ago.

Flat or Fisted Hands, Wedge or No Wedge:

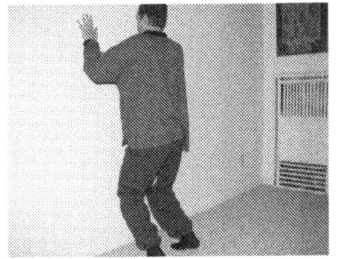 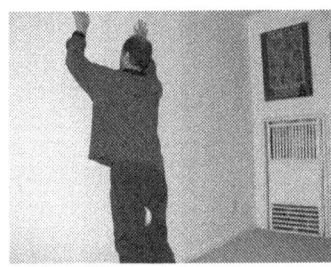

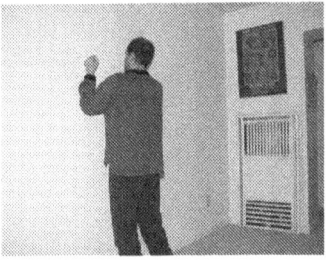

Go wild for a total body and aerobic workout. Up and down with your hands, flat or fisted. Bend your knees as you go down and straighten your legs on your way up. To stretch even higher, step up on your toes on your way up. Stay down for a while as you work with your hands and arms. To increase difficulty, try moving away or closer to the wall. Put on some loud music, have fun!

Use a mirror: stand in front of a full-length mirror to gauge how well you stand. If you find that your upper body is tilted over to your stronger leg, shift your weight back over to your weaker leg, and stay in the middle with both legs carrying the same load. Use muscles in your weaker leg and it will get stronger over time. Try to stay level whenever you are on your feet.

Cooling Down

After a satisfying routine, you feel invigorated. I find that to maintain a euphoric state long after the Agili Wellness Routine is performed, it is best to invest just a few more moments and conclude it gracefully. First, allow your body to come down, and then find your favorite and most comfortable position.

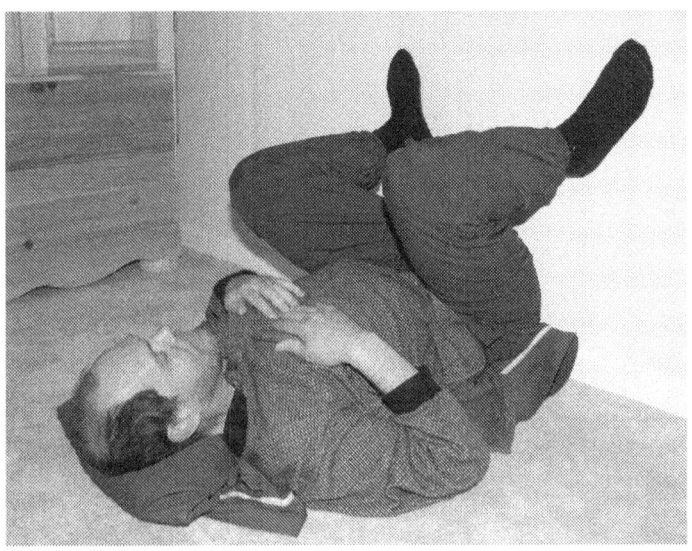

This is a good time to switch to a meaningful thought pattern, such as imagining a favorite place or experience, while bringing your awareness back to your breath for a few moments. Design a concluding and personal ritual that will send you off to your next activity with a healing and positive attitude. I sometimes use my favorite stretch during the final moments of the Agili Wellness Routine.

For comments or questions, use AgiliMail@aol.com.

Use the Agili Wellness Routine daily, and stay tuned for Book 2.

About the Author

Ofer Agam has been living with Multiple Sclerosis since 1974. After having tried many forms of physical activities and therapies for over a decade, he started formulating his own exercises. In 'The Agili Wellness Routine, Book 1', he shares how individuals with physical challenges or sedentary life style can greatly improve their lives through an effective daily routine that includes meditation and pragmatic exercises. Agam is working as a computer programmer for a non-profit organization, and is living in San Francisco Bay Area with his wife, two children and a cat called Sierra.

www.ingramcontent.com/pod-product-compliance
Lightning Source LLC
Chambersburg PA
CBHW050341290526

45785CB00006B/2584